The
New Mama Guide

Taking care of yourself in the first 6 weeks after birth

By
Jocelyn Lin

Maplekey Company
2015

Acknowledgements

A grateful thank-you goes to all who helped with the survey by spreading the word or generously sharing their experiences as first-time moms.

I'd like to also acknowledge the amazing feedback from my initial readers, who took the time and energy to send thoughtful comments and ideas: Angela, Seanna, Olga, Helena, Grace, Josh, Letitia, and Jane.

And, I owe my sister, whom I coerced into copy editing, when she would have preferred writing depressing literature in the wilds of Iowa.

Finally, thanks to my family, my guy, and the little pips for their support and love.

Table of contents

About this guide

During your pregnancy, you probably read a lot of books and got a lot of advice about caring for yourself through those nine months. You probably also learned how to prepare for the birth. In comparison, there is surprisingly little out there about what happens to you after the baby comes. Most information focuses entirely on the baby, and if you're lucky, you might find a couple pages in those pregnancy books about the medical after-effects of birth or phone numbers to call if you're feeling blue. What's up with that?!

This handbook is meant to fill in that knowledge gap by guiding you through what to expect from your new situation and body for the first 6 weeks after birth. It covers things that no one tells you because they're too embarrassed to say it or they're afraid of scaring you. And yeah, some of it is freaky, but it's even scarier to navigate this new terrain without the slightest clue.

For my first baby, I felt pretty good, and maybe a little smug going into my due date. I'd taken birth classes, stocked up on all the must-have nursery items, and read up on how to take care of a shiny new baby. Then … I got an unplanned c-section, which I didn't realize happens for 1 in 5 women. The surprises piled on from there, like my 2am hunger pangs with an empty pantry. And the very many hours a day just sitting and feeding the baby. And realizing that the vague warnings about not sleeping actually meant sleep deprivation torture! It was so tough to deal with all of this on top of caring for a newborn.

I wondered, why did nobody warn me exactly how hard it was going to be on myself? I could have at least prepared myself better for that difficult post-partum period. Later, when I felt more like myself and looked around, I couldn't find a single book on the subject. And so, I wrote this guide for you, so that your first 6 weeks with your little one can be a wonderful time (or at least less crappy!).

For this book, instead of relying on my experience alone, I surveyed 230 women about their post-birth experiences. Imagine hundreds of your closest, over-sharing girlfriends answering all sorts of questions about the first 6 weeks! You'll see later on that this information is collected into charts and statistics (like "1 in 4 women") to show you not only what's typical, but also how much outside "normal" you might end up being. Just remember — every mom and every baby is different, and that's ok!

Here's an example chart, and how to read it:

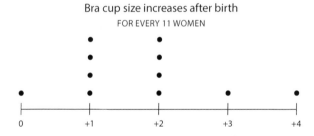

Bra cup size increases after birth
FOR EVERY 11 WOMEN

After birth, you can see that most (about 4 out of 5) women grow 1-2 cup sizes, but there are a few that stay the same or grow 3 or 4 sizes instead. So chances are that you'll grow 1-2 cup sizes, but then again, if you don't, you're certainly not alone.

For more information and tips, visit the companion website http://newmamaguide.com.

• • • • •

If you look outside of America, you'll find other cultures where postnatal practices celebrate and protect the new mother. For example, in much of East Asia, new moms are expected to devote the first month primarily to recuperation; there are special pampering clinics you can stay at, or often your mother-in-law stays to help out. Both Latin America and the Middle East institute a similar 40-day rest, with others doing housework and care. In the Netherlands, a kraamzorg comes by for a week after birth to offer professional postnatal maternity (and house!) care.

Did you find yourself drooling? America's family leave and support policies are far behind many other countries, and new moms are often expected to receive social visitors as soon they get home from the hospital. Many people also don't live near family, removing a primary source of help. We should be more supportive of new mamas! At the very least, you should take care of yourself and give yourself the gift of a good, healing first 6 weeks with your new baby.

• • • • •

A few side notes …
- The margins have been set extra wide so that you can scribble your own notes beside the text. Or if you're giving this book as a gift to a friend, use that space to add your personal tips.
- This guide devotes some space to breastfeeding because it's tricky and involves your body, but you should feel ok about feeding your baby however you want.
- There will be no mention of taking care of the baby at all, except from the perspective of how to work feeding and diaper-changing and other baby-care tasks into your new schedule. This book is about YOU. Baby-care is important, of course, but many books and websites out there cover that in great detail.
- Take the charts and numbers with a grain of salt. The survey responses are collected from my extended

Facebook network, which means that there is some sampling bias.

Introduction
What the heck just happened?

So … you've had your first baby! Good job, lady, and congratulations! You will soon notice that EVERYTHING is different now. It's truly amazing to have a new little one in your life. At the same time, many factors may contribute to making the period that follows one of the most challenging times of your life. For example:

- Your body needs to heal from pregnancy and birth — you CREATED another person!
- New, temporary, hormones are messing around with your emotions. Many people experience depression or the "baby blues" (cute name, not-cute experience).
- You have almost zero personal freedom and time. It's a very drastic shift from before.
- Oh yeah, and there's a baby living with you. Newborns need constant attention and care.

Sometimes, you'll be flying high and in love. But other times, you'll be miserable and lonely, and feel like your body isn't your own anymore.

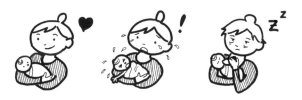

Try not to take things too seriously during this busy time. You'll get a lot of advice, but it's only advice. There's no right answer, so try not to stress too much. Ignore what others say if it makes you unhappy (excepting serious medical guidelines). Each person and each baby is different, so get a sense for what makes you feel nervous or comforted.

For me, some things that I stressed over for no reason were: tracking every single feeding as if I were a lab scientist, avoiding microwaving the milk, and not watching TV in front of the baby. The next time around, at least for the first 6 weeks, I am totally watching all the TV I want.

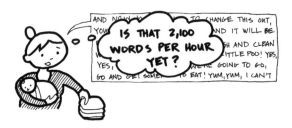

Above all, don't forget to take care of yourself. It's important for a baby to have a happy and healthy mama, too. So hang in there! It can be tough at first, but things change all the time, and it will be a fascinating experience watching your little one blossom and grow.

Chapter 1
The first 2-4 days.
Recovering from birth

Birth is a crazy experience, and it's a big change for your body after the previous months of pregnancy. Skip this chapter if you're squeamish (and read it in the hospital afterwards, when nothing could POSSIBLY make you squeamish anymore). Otherwise, on we go …

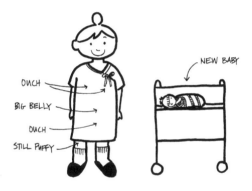

You'll still look pregnant. Sorry. Accept that now.

You probably already realized this with birth, but there is no such thing as modesty! I had nurses popping in at all hours trying to help me latch, a surprise visit from the infant hearing testers, a couple of check-ins from the pediatrician, and more. Of course, the visits were always perfectly timed so that people were walking in just as I was taking off all my clothes to attempt breastfeeding.

BODILY FUNCTIONS
Pooping
Ask for a stool softener right away, as they may not think to offer it, and take it regularly. Pooping is no fun, especially the first time after birth. Make sure to get some fiber in your diet.

Peeing
It can be intimidating if you got a catheter (which you will with an epidural). Everything gets swollen and numb so it feels more difficult than usual, but it's ok! It doesn't hurt when they take it out. The pee will eventually come out, and that won't hurt either.

Lochia: that thing that's like a period, but NOT AT ALL
You get something like a very heavy period, but it will look more like a grisly murder scene. It's gross, and it's messy, but only for the first few days. My nurses supplied disposable underwear and layered multiple maxi pads inside. Or you can try adult diapers. It's nice to not have to worry about the mess and laundry. This will taper quickly to something more like a regular period and reduce even more, eventually stopping after a couple weeks to a month for most people. You'll want to stock up on pads in advance.

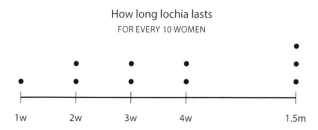

How long lochia lasts
FOR EVERY 10 WOMEN

1w   2w   3w   4w   1.5m

BIRTH AND MEDICAL PROCEDURES
Only 1 in every 10 people end up with a natural birth that has

no side effects or complications. For everyone else, you'll likely run into something that makes recovery take a little longer, ranging from 1st degree tears to something more serious.

Birth is very unpredictable, and it can be upsetting to face procedures you didn't expect, some of which occur surprisingly quickly. Keep in mind that the medical staff's number one priority is your and your baby's safety, so things are done for good reason. Here's what to expect and how to cope with different situations:

Vaginal birth (3 OUT OF 4 WOMEN)

The first poop is scary but ok. Tearing is quite common for your first birth because, well, geometry. Things that will help you feel better include:
- Ice packs
- Sitz baths
- Numbing spray
- Tucks medicated pads
- Maxi pads soaked in witch hazel and stored in the freezer
- Soft cushions or a donut pillow to sit on

Tears and episiotomies (1 OUT OF 2 VAGINAL BIRTHS)

It will hurt to sit, and the pain will likely last a few weeks, though to heal completely, it can take months (especially for episiotomies and serious tears). An unlucky few get both tears and an episiotomy. You may have these even with an unplanned cesarean, depending on how far along things got before you needed a c-section after all. That really sucks! Some more things that will help you feel better include:
- Soft cushions or a donut pillow to sit on
- Keeping things clean down there
  Drink and pee a lot, rinsing with a squirt bottle after each trip to the bathroom.

Tear and episiotomy occurrence
FOR EVERY 10 VAGINAL BIRTHS

episiotomies ● ○ ○ ○ ○ ○ ○ ○ ○ ○

tears ⊕ ⊘ ⊘ ● ● ○ ○ ○ ○ ○

1°   2°   3°

Hemorrhoids

You can get this with both vaginal and c-section deliveries. It will hurt to poop and it may be uncomfortable sitting. Things that will help you feel better:

- Stool softeners
- Creams or medications that will help relieve pain and swelling (ask your doctor)

Swelling/ edema

Your body has extra blood and fluids that you made during pregnancy (also from any IVs you had during delivery), so you might swell up afterwards.

It doesn't hurt, it's just uncomfortable. You'll get rid of it after a week or so of sweating and many extra trips to the bathroom. There's not much you can do, except for avoiding overly salty food so that you don't retain fluids. Note that if it actually hurts or is worse on one side, that's a different (rare) problem; call your doctor right away.

Cesareans (1 OUT OF 4 BIRTHS)

There are the pre-scheduled and then there are the unplanned cesareans. 1 out of every 5 women who go into the delivery room for a vaginal birth end up with an unplanned c-section. (That was me, surprise!)

It will hurt to laugh or cough for the first few days, since you had serious abdominal surgery. Your incision will likely be just below the bikini line. You can't sit up easily, so pull yourself up with your arms or roll over off the bed. You also won't be able to walk around easily for a few days. Things that may help you feel better:

- Small pillow for holding against your incision
- Belly band to hold things in
- Not picking up anything heavy
- Taking short walks down the hall

And so on …

About 1 in 10 people experience other issues. Sadly, it's not uncommon to run into infections, incontinence, or bowel problems. Less common, serious problems may occur related to bleeding, preeclampsia, or sepsis (an infection complication marked by fevers). It's hard to prepare for these things, but if you'd like to learn more, some pregnancy books, such as the What to Expect series, cover these contingencies.

RECOVERY

How quickly you bounce back from birth really depends on your body and what happened. The next page shows how long it took for various people to sit, stand, and walk again without too much trouble. Likely, it took longer to feel 100%.

Sadly, American hospitals and insurance send you back home after just 2 days, so make sure you have the right environment and support at home to continue healing. You may also go home with a prescription, so have someone available to run to the pharmacist for you.

The first medical follow up usually happens a whopping 6 weeks later. This is a very long time to resolve issues, especially if you had surgical procedures done. You won't know what feels abnormal (EVERYTHING!) so do call in with every little question you may have in the meantime.

How long before feeling sort-of-ok after birth
FOR EVERY 10-11 WOMEN, PER PROCEDURE

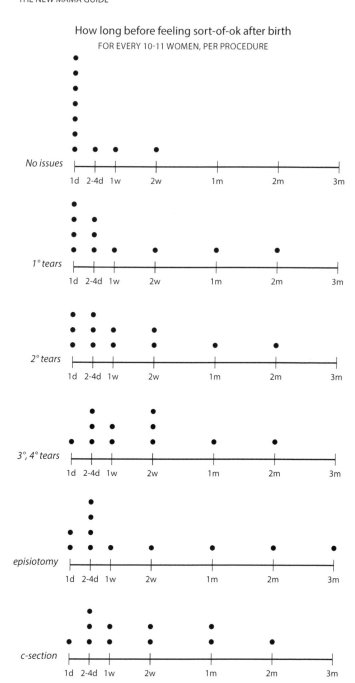

YOUR BODY

Again, yes, you'll still look pregnant after giving birth! And, your boobs will probably grow, sometimes an astounding amount. You'll probably be about the same shape as you were at 5-7 months pregnant, and grow one or two cup sizes from before pregnancy.

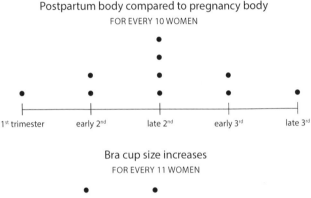

Postpartum body compared to pregnancy body
FOR EVERY 10 WOMEN

1st trimester   early 2nd   late 2nd   early 3rd   late 3rd

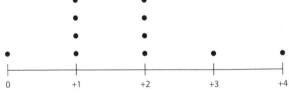

Bra cup size increases
FOR EVERY 11 WOMEN

0   +1   +2   +3   +4

What to wear

They give you a gown at the hospital, which is pretty convenient. If you plan to breastfeed, bring along a super stretchy nursing bra as your boobs figure things out and settle in size. A belly band or binder might help you feel more together, but some don't care for those. Try a soft, stretchy one so you can sit while wearing it without anything digging into your body.

Go home in your maternity clothes. If you had a relatively uneventful birth, then the yoga pants are fine. Otherwise, stay away from pants and try a stretch knit skirt with a nursing top, or better yet, something that doesn't touch your bottom half at all, like a dress. Also, having cheap grandma panties on hand is useful, especially if you got a c-section. (Your incision will thank you for having a waistband up by your belly button, instead of rubbing against it at the bikini line.)

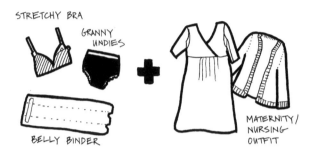

Taking care of yourself supply checklist

- Rinsing bottle thing
- Soft pillow or donut pillow to sit on
- Ice packs/ sitz baths/ numbing spray/ witch hazel pads
- Small pillow to hold over your incision if you had a c-section
- If you breastfeed, cream or soothing cold gel pads. See also: Breastfeeding Tips, Chapter 11.
- Belly band

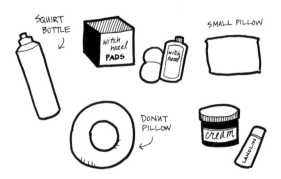

Chapter 2
The first week: goodbye to sleep, what does it mean?

When people tell you that you won't sleep anymore, what does it mean? Well, for the first day, your baby is really tired after the ordeal and might be sleepy. You should sleep, too. Once they start getting hungry, though, they are hungry ALL THE TIME! No more delicious undisturbed sleep for you!

TIMING

You must feed and change the baby at least every 2-3 hours, and likely more often at times. Note that the 2-3 hours include the time it takes to actually nurse and diaper. THIS is why sleep is so difficult.

Each feeding will take 20-45 min at first. They are slow and you have to actively help the baby eat because they are like a floppy sack of flour.

You won't get more than 3 consecutive hours of sleep. Sometimes, you'll get only 1 hour because it took you 15 minutes of lying there to fall asleep yourself, and then the baby inconveniently gets hungry only 2 hours after the beginning of the last feeding. Or, maybe the baby decided to cluster feed at 4am. Argh!

Newborns often get their nights and days all messed up. You may be up alone with the baby for long stretches in the middle of the night. This schedule is exhausting, especially if you can't nap during the day because of other responsibilities.

It's really hard to be sleep-deprived. Take every chance you have to try to sleep. It's ok if you're just closing your eyes; at least that's better than staying awake and bustling about.

You've probably heard this one, but the number one tip people like to give and receive is: "Sleep while the baby sleeps." I really grew to hate hearing that, because it is both true and hard to follow. It is hard to avoid the surprisingly strong urge to spend baby sleep time as me-downtime (like surfing social networks on your phone) or on doing household chores. And inevitably, the people telling you this are all bright-eyed and bushy-tailed with plenty of sleep, and you just kind of want to smack them.

To give you a better picture, here's an example schedule for when you and your newborn eat and sleep (assuming that you need to be awake whenever your baby is and that you'd like to shower each day). By the way, don't expect little ones to follow a real schedule, this is just a sense of how often they need to be taken care of.

Sample sleeping and eating schedule for just you and your newborn

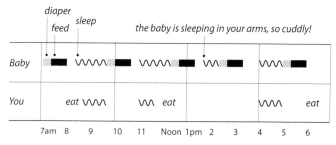

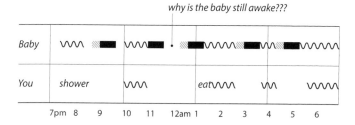

Now imagine doing this every single day for weeks on end. It's like torture!

TIPS

- Use bottles, even if you breastfeed
  This means that someone else can feed the baby while you sleep. Even once a day or once every few days can make a big difference.
- Find a baby sleep book that fits your style
  Read up on baby waking and sleep cycles, so you know what to expect and can plan your own schedule around that.
- Nurse in a safe place
  You will be very tired and might fall asleep while nursing. Try to position yourself and your baby so that if it happens, your baby won't fall anywhere dangerous.

Hang in there!

After a while, babies get much better at latching on and quicker at eating. They wait longer between meals and start consolidating their sleep, which all adds up to more time and more sleep for you later on. So know that it's not forever, and hang in there!

Here's where the light at the end of the tunnel might fall:

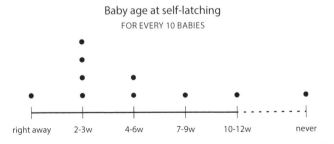

Baby age at self-latching
FOR EVERY 10 BABIES

right away   2-3w   4-6w   7-9w   10-12w   never

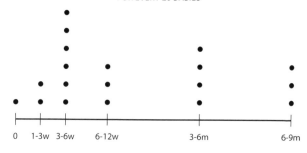

Baby age when feeding time drops below 30 minutes
FOR EVERY 20 BABIES

That first time the baby sleeps more than 3 hours in a row will feel really good. (But instead of taking advantage of the extra time, you'll probably end up checking every 10 minutes to see if the baby is still breathing.)

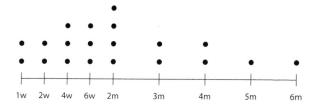

Baby age at first 3+ hours of consecutive sleep
FOR EVERY 20 WOMEN

This will likely happen by 1-2 months. Note that your baby will also have less frequent feedings over time.

• • • • •

The first time you get to sleep more than 3 hours in a row will feel amazing (also probably by 1-2 months).

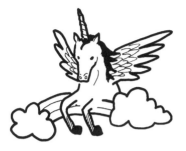

Baby age at YOUR first 3+ hours of consecutive sleep
FOR EVERY 20 WOMEN

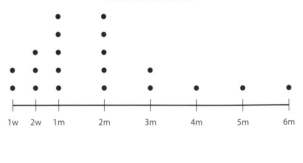

• • • • •

When you finally get to regularly sleep more than 3 hours in a row, it will feel like you won the lottery and a lifetime supply of chocolate croissants.

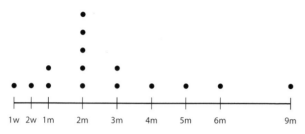

Baby age when you regularly get 3+ hours of consecutive sleep
FOR EVERY 20 WOMEN

You can do it!

Chapter 3
Recovering at home, what to eat

You need to nourish your body so that it can replenish itself. If you happen to be nursing as well, you'll be starving all the time and very thirsty. Don't ignore that! You'll need to take in additional fuel and nutrients to create magical milk for your baby. Drink tons of water, too.

WHAT KIND OF FOOD?

- Hot and nourishing
  "Healthy" things like cold carrot sticks and almonds won't leave you feeling satisfied.
- Easy to reheat and eat quickly
  Especially when you're starving and hanging out with a wide-awake infant by yourself in the middle of the night.
- Easy to open and eat with one hand
  In case you're the only one around and you're holding a fussy baby (granola bar wrappers, for example, are not easy to open one-handed).

Make lots of easy-to-reheat meals in advance, at least 2 weeks' worth, if not 1-2 months' worth, depending on how much outside help you will be getting with meals.

SPECIFIC EXAMPLES

- Nothing too spicy or salty
  Some people get tummy upsets from spicy food or find that salty foods make swelling worse early on.
- Meat-based brothy soups
  These are great because they keep you hydrated and full of nutrition. They're also easier to digest in the first few days.
  - · Chicken, vegetable, and rice soup with an entire chicken in there
  - · Minestrone with meatballs
  - · Asian noodle soups with any meat (pork, beef, shrimp, fish cakes) and baby bok choy
  - · Tip: Keep a soup thermos ready for one-handed eating/drinking
- Hot, filling stuff
- Meat and potatoes
  - · Curry and rice
  - · Roast chicken and root vegetables
- Food that you can make and freeze in advance
  - · Soup, chilies, and stews
  - · Meatballs, hamburger patties, meatloaves
  - · Roast or grilled chicken
  - · Casseroles
  - · Burritos
  - · Muffins and breads

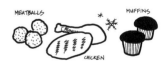

- Food that is easy to throw together
  - · Stew made in the slow cooker, using pre-chopped grocery veggies and stew meats

· Couscous from a box + zapped frozen veggies + thawed meatballs
· Spaghetti with jarred sauce
· Instant oatmeal in the microwave with raisins and milk
· Peanut butter sandwich + banana
· Eggs

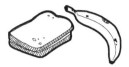

• Emergency food for when you really have no time
  · Prepared frozen dinners
    (I personally found frozen Chinese dumplings to be tasty, healthy, and filling)
  · Low-sodium canned soups + bread

Remember those cultures that nurture mothers after birth? Here are some traditional dishes that they make for the new mom to eat:

• Korea: miyeok-guk, seaweed soup + rice
• Mexico: hot chocolate or atole, a hot corn-milkshake-like drink
• Lebanon: m'jurda, rice and lentils
• Taiwan: ma you ji, sesame oil chicken + rice (but skip the rice wine)
• Saudi Arabia: lamb soup
• China: pig's feet and peanut soup

SNACKS AND DRINKS

Keep fatty, protein-rich snacks on hand for random hunger attacks or if a meal won't be ready anytime soon. Try stashing little caches around the house in strategic areas, including by your bed. Snack ideas:

• String cheese and Babybels

- Peanuts and cashews
- Trail mix
- Cookies, protein bars, and granola bars
- Dried fruit, like prunes and apricots
- Low-sodium beef jerky

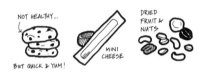

Keep water on hand. Use a container that won't leak and has a flip top that can be operated one-handed. Ideally, it's also clear so that you can see whether it needs refills.

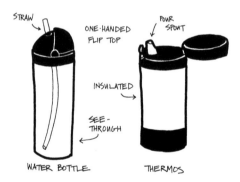

Chapter 4
Feeding a baby is wonderful but also incredibly boring

It's true that feeding your snuggly little bundle is a lovely bonding moment. They're happily nursing away while you look at their teeny noses and gaze soulfully into their eyes. But …

There is nothing else to do while feeding them, and there is only so much gazing you can do for 7 hours a day, every day. Your smartphone, eBook reader, laptop, or TV will become your best friend in the early months. What you can do depends on how many hands you have free.

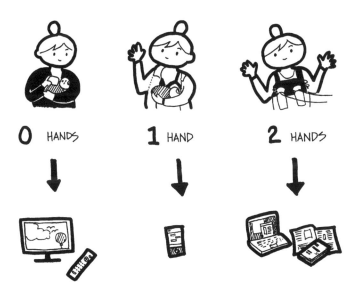

Things to stock up on and do:
- Silly feel-good novels and magazines
- Helpful baby books
- Addictive TV series on DVD, Hulu, or Netflix
  Tip: Avoid anything sad or with unhappy children. I found that my crazy hormones made me sob at any hint of kids being hurt.
- Video or phone games
  Especially ones where you won't lose if you put it down in the middle.
- Anything easy to pick up and put down right away

After talking to some friends, I found out that I wasn't the only one who avoided watching shows due to a sense of guilt. There's an official pediatrician guideline about not letting children younger than 2 watch TV. But (too late) I realized that tiny babies are blobs that can't see past the distance of your face, so for the first few weeks, at least, it's not like they can see the TV anyway. As with everything, though, it's up to you!

Chapter 5
Recovering at home, what else to do

Take it easy as much as you can. Take care of yourself and the baby first before you take care of the house. Sleeping and eating for yourself should take up most of your non-baby time.

PERSONAL HYGIENE

It will feel like you can't put the baby down for a moment, but you can! Taking care of yourself will make such a big difference in how you feel.

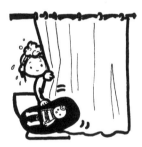

Tips:
- Put your baby in a bouncer or swing while you take care of yourself and other necessities, if no one else is available to take them.
- Try to take a hot shower every day. If you actually manage that, you're doing great! If not, that's totally normal.
- Stock up on facial wipes.
- Brush your teeth at least once a day, but don't worry about eating right afterwards if your schedule doesn't work out.

- Give yourself a fun pedicure now that you can see your toes again.
- You won't have much time to deal with contacts if you wear them, so make sure to update your glasses prescription beforehand.

ENTERTAINMENT AND HOBBIES

To keep sane, find new things that can fit into small increments of time.

Ideas:
- Read those baby books you got or browse the internet for guides and tips. Take advice with a grain of salt.
- Knitting or crocheting is an excellent activity when things are less of a blur, because you can do very small bits in your random 3 minutes here and there.
- Go out and get some air for a mood booster. It doesn't matter where, it doesn't even matter if it's just standing outside the door for a few minutes — just do it.

Holding a small baby takes up one arm. Many activities will need adapting to be one-handed. If your baby tolerates it, try baby-wearing so you can do things while holding them. And, as mentioned earlier, there are bouncers and swings you can put your baby into as well.

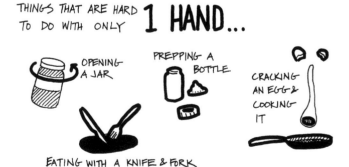

THINGS THAT ARE HARD TO DO WITH ONLY **1 HAND...**

OPENING A JAR

PREPPING A BOTTLE

CRACKING AN EGG & COOKING IT

EATING WITH A KNIFE & FORK

Chapter 6
Help: partner support

If you have a partner, good support can improve a mom's wellbeing. This can be a life partner or a very close relative or friend staying to help out. Ideally, your partner will make it easier for you to concentrate on recuperating. If your partner works outside the home, see if they can take parental leave to help you out for those first few weeks, especially if you had a tough time with birth and/or don't have other help coming by.

Once the baby is here, take turns with your partner at being the primary caretaker of the baby and being the expert at some task. Don't feel like you're the only one who can do everything. It will lessen the load for you and help your partner start developing a closer bond with the baby.

WHO DOES WHAT

It's also a good idea to establish "jobs" from the beginning. For example, if you're the only one that can do feedings, then your partner is the one that picks up the baby and does diaper changes. Share the pain of waking up at 4am! Here are some examples of things only you can do versus things that you can both do (and which your partner can therefore take over).

Things only you can do
- Breastfeed or pump (7+ hours per day)

Things either of you can do, but your partner should if you're nursing or pumping
- Hold the baby while they're plain old awake (2 hours)
- Soothe the baby to sleep (depends on baby fussiness)
- Change diapers (2 hours)

- Do housework: Meals, dishes, laundry, etc. (2-3 hours)
- Bottle-feed the baby (depends)
- Bathe baby (a few times a week)
- Communicate to other people how to help

If this looks overwhelming, remember that these numbers are for newborns! Things are different after a few weeks and even more so after a few months.

Remember that daily sleep and activity schedule for you and your baby from Chapter 1? Here's a new version with suggestions on how to fit both your and your partner's essential activities in.

Sample schedule for you, a partner there all day, and a newborn

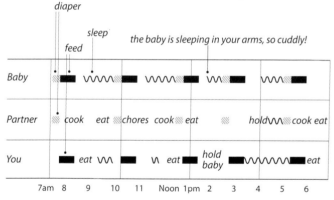

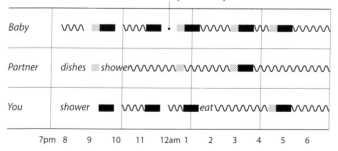

Check the appendix for a blank version if you'd like to customize it or add other helpers. The newmamaguide.com website has a printable download that you can also use.

LIFE PARTNERS: COMMUNICATION

There is now an amazing new little one in your lives, which makes the two of you into three. It's a big change! Sometimes, you'll all lie there together and bask in happy baby glow, examining tiny baby hands. And those little yawns! And those very edible-looking teeny baby feet!

But, once in a while, there may be not-so-great feelings, perhaps even moments of resentment. This can happen even with the best and most helpful partner ever, especially if you're nursing or pumping. (In this case, you're getting much less sleep than your partner and the baby depends that much more on just you. Resentment city.)

Hash out all of this before you give birth, while you are both still well rested and sane. Fortunately, today's partners are much more involved than they were a generation ago; 3 out of 5 new moms with partners have very supportive ones, while 1 out of 5 have partners unable to help for some reason. If you sense that your partner might not be as supportive as needed, don't hesitate to ask for more help or to turn to friends and family.

In general, check in on each other once in a while, even if you are both exhausted. Compliment each other. Having a newborn is tough on any relationship. Be very precise about your needs and wants; for example, say, "Please hold the baby for 15 minutes while I go to the bathroom." No one can read your mind!

However easy or tough it is, nothing beats watching your relationship evolve from a couple into a family.

LIFE PARTNERS: SEXY TIMES

Different people wait different amounts of time before they have sex again. It depends on your situation and how you're recovering. Many people go for it within the first 3-6 months, but for some, it can take up to 1 or 2 years to get in the mood again.

Know that breastfeeding hormones will negatively affect your desire for, and comfort with, sexy times. It can take around a month or so after you stop nursing for that effect to go away. If you don't want kids again in the near future, don't forget your birth control (and lubrication)! Talk to your doctor before you get started again, to make sure everything's ship-shape and to know what your options are.

Chapter 7
Help: things that others can do

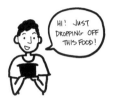

Remember, you're supposed to be healing and restoring your body in the first 6 weeks. You shouldn't be doing any work outside of sleeping, resting, and feeding the baby, and that's where other people come in. Take all the good help you can get, especially if they're volunteering food.

You don't want to be stuck playing host to houseguests or even visitors while you're trying to get better! Avoid social visitors for the first 6 weeks (unless that sort of thing energizes you), don't invite too many people ahead of time, and play it by ear after the baby comes. If people really want to come, have them bring food as the price of admission for seeing you and the baby.

The best kind of helper listens to your instructions and doesn't make any demands. This can be awkward to tell family, and much easier to deal with in hired help. Unfortunately, not all of us are lucky enough to be able to afford a regular caretaker.

USEFUL THINGS HELPERS CAN DO
- Providing warm, fuzzy feelings and emotional support
- Doing housework, like dishes, laundry, and cleaning
- Buying groceries and food
- Cooking meals

- Bringing food in disposable containers
- Holding your baby while you shower, go to the bathroom, or sleep
- Giving tips on diaper changing techniques and other practical advice

NOT USEFUL

- Chitchatting when you are tired and want to sleep
- Making you feel like you need to clean and look good for visits
- Giving advice that you do not want or need
- Saying that your opinions and wishes are wrong

PARENTS AND IN-LAWS

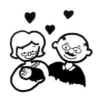

They can be amazingly supportive and helpful, and 2 out of 4 new moms who had them visit say they can't do without them. But know that you tend to hear about the wonderful ones, because people are reluctant to say unkind things about their own parents or in-laws. The truth is that 1 in 4 new moms with grandparent visitors had very stressful ones! That's a lot!

All the guidelines for helpful visitors also apply to grandparents. It's great if they help take care of the housework, hold the baby, and give you emotional support. These gestures are especially invaluable if you don't have a partner or your partner isn't able to pull his or her weight. On the other hand, it can be stressful to have a critical authority figure hovering around while you're trying to figure things out and do what you think is best. Things were also done differently a generation ago, and it's hard to argue back when someone tells you that you or your partner turned out just fine with their methods.

It's so important for you and your baby's health and happiness not to bring extra stress into your first few months. The survey this book is based on shows a correlation between quality of support and mom's mental well-being. So here's a quick quiz to ask yourself and your partner:

Does being around them comfort and relax both of you?	YES NO
Would you ask them for advice on big life decisions? (Ex: buying a car, careers, serious health issues)	YES NO
Are they ok with their advice or opinions not being followed?	YES NO
Are they ok with you having your own opinions and methods?	YES NO
Are you willing to support each other by standing up to your own parents if needed? (Standing up to in-laws doesn't work!)	YES NO

If all the answers are yes, then invite them! For weeks and weeks! Just make sure that both of you get enough bonding time with baby, as a very helpful grandparent may unintentionally make one of you feel left out.

If any answers are no, then discuss and think about it more seriously. If you don't want them to come in the first 6 weeks, it's very hard to tell them no, but someone does have to put their foot down. And, in this case, the new mama should get the final say.

Chapter 8
Housework

Avoid as much housework as possible in the first 6 weeks —
you should be recovering! This is where well-intentioned helpers
can best be put to work. If you can afford it, hiring help is
great, even just once a month, and there's no question that the
more budget you have, the easier it is.

You will read and hear a lot of advice that tells you not to stress
about dirty dishes or floors. And it is ok to not sweep the floor
or clean the bathroom for a few weeks. But frankly, it gets
pretty gross after that, and SOMEONE needs to do something.
And that someone might be you.

If you end up having to do it yourself after all, here are some
things to stock up on:
- Disposable everything
- Swiffers and Clorox wipes
  Don't bother with reusable rags and mops. And make
  sure you DO NOT confuse household cleaner wipes
  with the diaper wipes!
- Disposable dishes and silverware to avoid washing
- Disposable paper towels
- Disposable diapers until you're settled into the routine
  Even if you're planning on cloth diapering, there's no
  sense making it harder on yourself in those hectic first
  6 weeks.
- Contact info for delivery services that will bring things
  to you
  These can be ones for anything from groceries
  (Safeway) to diapers (Google shopping or Amazon) to
  prepared food, or ones that will run your errands
  (TaskRabbit).

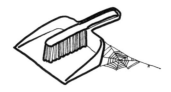

Unfortunately, I don't have many tips for avoiding sweeping, vacuuming, and laundry, as they all actually have to be done. Adjust your standards and pace. It's ok to sweep just one part of the room at a time, whenever you have a spare minute. There's no need to clean an entire room at once. And it's ok to just leave clean piles of laundry on the couch instead of neatly folding it up and putting it away — hey, at least you managed to get it clean.

Chapter 9
Feeeeelings

It's pretty common to have moments where you feel down. New hormones are coursing through you, and massive changes have happened to your body and your lifestyle.

Your mood very much depends on your personality and your particular situation. It can be anywhere from all sunshine to all clouds. People who are blissfully happy with blinding amounts of baby love (1 out of 10 of you) should skip to the next chapter right now!

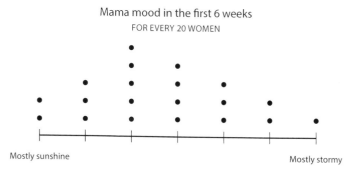

Mama mood in the first 6 weeks
FOR EVERY 20 WOMEN

Mostly sunshine   Mostly stormy

For the rest of us, a whole range of factors can contribute to feelings of isolation and stress, such as:
- The sudden change in personal freedom
  You're going from absolute freedom to caring for a helpless newborn 24/7. Days can be quite long and you can feel lonely and like you have no sense of self anymore.
- Intense hormonal feelings
- Feeling like your body is not your own anymore
  There's a baby and perhaps a partner touching and making demands of it, all day long.

- Feeling like you've failed because birth and nursing didn't match up to ideals
- Medical complications from birth
  The healing process isn't always easy or quick.
- Breastfeeding or pumping, which can take its toll
- Less helpful partners or parents
- Babies who have reflux, colic, or other issues
- Just because (there doesn't have to be a reason)

You may feel very alone sometimes and randomly cry. It might also be difficult to bond with the baby right away, especially if there are other stressors. It's all normal, and you're actually not alone! As you can see from the chart above, it's very common for new moms to go through a funk. Find a non-judgmental mom group online or in person to vent to, and know that it gets much, much better. If it gets bad, or if you find it hard to care anymore, then please talk to a professional.

If you are doing something that makes you unhappy, evaluate whether you can stop — being a new mama doesn't mean being a martyr! Some pieces of advice prioritize baby over mama, and it's often perfectly okay to go a different route.

Also remember that there are many moments to treasure, with a lovely smelling, snuggly, cute baby. The bad feelings won't last forever. Here's a big hug { }. You'll be ok!

Chapter 10
What's going on with your milk-producing boobs

If you're not breastfeeding or pumping (totally ok!), skip ahead to Chapter 15.

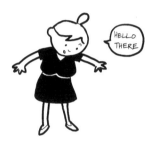

So you've read up on how beneficial breast milk is for babies, and you've decided to give it a go. Great! It's cheaper and also much more convenient to be able to pull out a boob in the middle of the night, or while you're out at a restaurant, instead of worrying about bottles and formulas and temperature and washing up.

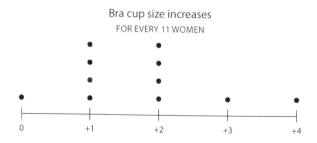

Bra cup size increases
FOR EVERY 11 WOMEN

Your boobs are probably going to get pretty big, growing 1-2 cup sizes on average. It's a great time to try boob-y outfits if you were small before, and learn how to dress a larger bust so that you don't get uniboob. But if you were already big, make sure they get very, VERY good support.

LETDOWN

Having milk rush into your body feels odd at first. For some it's painful (anywhere from prickles and needles to electrocution) and for some it's not. At first, engorgement is also quite common (6 out of 10 women) while your boobs are trying to figure out supply and demand. This is when you fill up too much, too quickly, and get rock hard breasts that need to be emptied. It's not comfortable. Your baby can take off the pressure for you, though it can be more difficult to latch onto something hard, or you can pump off the extra.

Once your body adjusts, within a couple days to a couple weeks, letdown becomes a very normal and non-painful part of your nursing routine.

Interestingly, it can happen with various triggers, like touch or hearing your baby cry. I found it fascinatingly weird that just thinking about feeding my baby made milk come in.

LEAKING

With an overactive letdown, you will also leak. This might be anything from a dribble to actual milk spraying out, which is as ridiculous as it sounds.

Tips to deal with heavier leaking (so that you don't have sour-smelling milk-crusted clothes all the time):
- As the baby feeds on one side, stuff the other side with towels.
- At home, stuff washable pads in your bra so that you have time to run for a washcloth when leaking.

- When going out, use the disposable kind. They have diaper technology! I personally found the washable ones to be too visible through clothes, and anyway, they tended to leak right through.

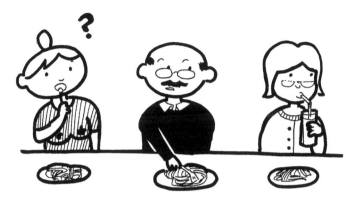

Imagine sitting down to dinner with your family and having drops of milk start leaking out through all of your clothes in front of your dad. Awkward! Not that this happened to me or anything.

Chapter 11
Breastfeeding tips

Know that breastfeeding and pumping are NOT easy at first. Both you and the baby are trying to figure things out together. It's about as natural as learning to ride a bike. All those beautiful soft focus photos you see of mothers and newborns happily attached? Bah! What they don't show you is all that went on beforehand: squeezing your nipple into the right shape, coaxing the baby to open its mouth, and trying to cram things in at the exact right second.

LACTATION CONSULTANTS

I highly recommend finding a good lactation consultant before you give birth. They are awesome. Don't ignore problems or hope they'll go away after a bit. Find one you like that matches your style. For example, if you are not sure that you want to keep up with breastfeeding, don't get one that will make you feel guilty about it.

Before you give birth, set up 2 visits in advance: once for immediately after delivery to learn the basics, and then again in 2 weeks to check in and adjust technique. You won't know what you're doing wrong.

Unfortunately, LCs may not be covered by insurance, and they can be expensive. You can also look into your local La Leche League for advice and help.

LATCHING PAIN

At the beginning, latching can really hurt! Your poor nipples aren't used to constant pressure and friction. Again, how much it hurts and how long it lasts depends on the individual person and baby. Sometimes, this can be caused by improper latching, so you'll need to adjust that.

For most people, it gets better by two weeks or else they call it quits with breastfeeding. Incredibly persistent folks might stick it out for 2-4 months, but that is not common, and frankly, I can't imagine being in pain for that long. And then, for some, the baby never latches properly, and that ends breast-feeding as well.

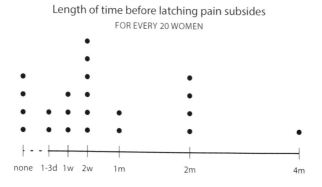

Length of time before latching pain subsides
FOR EVERY 20 WOMEN

To give yourself some relief, try applying cold gel pads, lanolin ointment, or Motherlove nipple cream.

Only you can judge how much you're willing to deal with and still be able to function properly. If it doesn't stop hurting, or if there are problems with the baby's latch, or it's just plain making you miserable, it's totally ok to move on. Your baby will be just fine on formula. If you want to keep trying, that's ok, too. These are your boobs, and you get to decide what to do with them.

WHAT TO WEAR AT HOME
It took me a couple weeks of shivering in the chilly 4am air

without a shirt on to figure out how to pop out just a boob and keep the rest of myself covered up and warm. Eventually, I found myself constantly in a comfortable uniform at home that made nursing easy. Here is what worked for me:

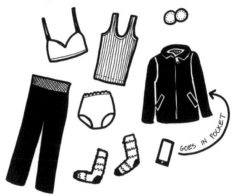

- Comfy nursing bra
  Once my size settled down, I liked the clippy ones best, since they're easy to operate one-handed.
- Ribbed knit tank top
  It's super stretchy for your giant boobs, but will stay put if you pull it up, so you're not trying to wrestle with baby, boob, pillows, AND clothes.
- Nursing camisole or tank
  In this case you don't need a separate tank top
- Zippered jacket, of the velour or sweatshirt kind
  This keeps your arms and back warm while your torso is exposed. Having a big zip-up pocket is even better so that you have somewhere to put your precious, precious smartphone. No hoodie, because that gets lumpy when you sleep in it.
- Washable leak-proof breast pads

HANDY SUPPLIES

Here are some useful things to keep on a table by your bed during those midnight wakeup calls.

- Pencil + paper for taking notes
- Not-too-bright lamp to see in the middle of the night
- Hearty snacks, for you will be very hungry
- Water to drink, for you will be very thirsty
- Small light-up analog clock that you can see in the wee hours, so you can quickly decide whether that 4am fussing means hunger (because your baby last ate at 1am) or a diaper change (because the last feeding was 3am). Personally, I found an analog clock much better than a digital one. It was just too hard to do the math with a digital clock when groggy, and easier to estimate how much time passed on an analog clock.

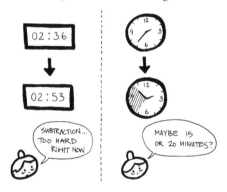

I'd also keep an extra set of these items by your preferred nursing or pumping spot, with the addition of some entertainment options and washcloths for cleanup.

ERGONOMICS ARE IMPORTANT

Some people swear by special pillows, some just use regular ones, and some have special chairs. It's different for each person, so try things out at the store or at your friends' houses. It's worth investing in up front, given the amount of time you spend nursing or feeding. Holding yourself in uncomfortable positions for extended periods of time can do bad things to your body.

At first, I thought these were just gadgets sold to gullible new parents and didn't bother with them. Months of breastfeeding later, I finally bought a nice chair and totally regretted the unnecessary aches and pains I put myself through earlier.

To make sure you're properly comfortable, you first want to make sure you're not exerting effort to hold up any part of baby. You'll tire quickly during the (20-40 minute!) session, and if you keep it up, you might get repetitive stress issues. This means that your pillow and chair arm should help prop up your arms and baby to boob level without you having to lift a muscle.

You should also be sitting comfortably in a good posture, which means sitting up straight, all the way back in your chair. Many typical armchairs are designed for lounging, so if you sit all the way back, your knees can't bend and you can't reach the arms comfortably at the same time. Nursing chairs are designed differently. I'm a short person (5'3"), so I had to try out many nursing chairs before I found one that fit my body properly.

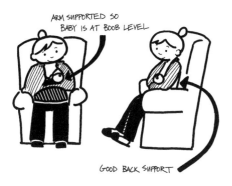

ARM SUPPORTED SO BABY IS AT BOOB LEVEL

GOOD BACK SUPPORT

If you have short legs like me, and they're left dangling, something to prop up your feet so your knees can rest at a 90-degree angle is also nice. A fancy nursing chair ottoman will do the job, as will stacking up diaper boxes with a towel for padding on top.

Chapter 12
Pumping tips

There are many reasons you might pump. For one, it lets you leave the house without the baby, either for short errands or for longer travel. Unfortunately, with the length of most American maternity leaves, pumping is a must if you want to continue feeding the baby breast milk after you go back to work.

You may also unexpectedly have to exclusively pump if you are committed to feeding breast milk and the baby is early or cannot latch. This takes a lot of time and can be lonely, so think about putting your home setup somewhere that allows you to still be a part of the family.

Research which pump is right for you, and have the parts clean and ready before birth. It's also a good idea to do a dry run to familiarize yourself with how the machine works and where everything goes. You're going to spend a lot of time attached to that thing and having a love-hate relationship with it. It will be unglamorous and make you feel like a cow. But on the bright side, it is a provider of life-sustaining miracle food for your baby!

SUPPLIES
- Pump and related plastic pieces
  Having 2 sets allows you to keep washing to a minimum or stash an extra set elsewhere.
- Large gallon Ziploc baggie
  Refrigerate your pump supplies in-between so that you only have to do one big washing a day.

- Sanitizing microwavable bags
  Instead of a regular baggie, you can refrigerate and then rinse and nuke your pump supplies in the special bags once a day.
- Bin of warm sudsy water + bottle brush for washing up
- Pumping bra
  Wear this over your clothes, like in the illustration below, so there's no need to take everything else off first. You can also try cutting holes into an old saggy bra or sports bra, or just shove the flanges into your stretchy nursing bra and brace them in with an arm.

HOME PUMPING STATION SETUP

Similar to the bedside and nursing list on page 47, you want your setup to be comfortable, entertaining, and hold all the supplies you need.

- Table to hold pump
- Comfy chair
- TV or laptop for entertainment
- Pumping bra
- Washcloths, tissues, or wipes to clean up
- Small bin holding clean pump supplies
- Hearty snacks and water to drink

PUMPING AWAY FROM HOME

Here are a few supplies you'll need if you are pumping away from your home setup.

- Containers to store milk, such as:
  - Baby bottles
    You'll probably need to buy the matching screw-on storage cap separately.
  - Milk storage bag and a sharpie for labeling
    You can lay the bags flat and freeze, then stack for easy storage in the freezer.
  - Glass stackable mason jars
- Large gallon Ziploc baggie
  This allows you to put pumping supplies into the fridge between sessions so that you can wash up once after you get home.
- Discreet insulated lunch bag with an ice pack
  Put your milk containers inside to store in a shared fridge and/or carry between locations

PUMPING AT WORK

At work, you also need to consider wearing clothes that make it easy to access your chest without taking off everything. So button-downs are good, while zip-up sheath dresses are not so smart. Bring a drink of water with you into the mother's room, as you'll get thirsty in there.

A basic setup for a mother's room includes:
- Table
- Fridge
- Big mirror for checking yourself before going back to work
- Chair
- Outlet for pump
- Paper towels
- Trash can
- Lock on door

A great setup would also include a sink and drying rack for cleaning up and some sort of white noise, like a fan, so that people nearby can't hear the pump. While we're dreaming, let's add an extra pump that stays at the office.

If you don't have an accommodating workplace with a dedicated pumping space, then you will need to find an available lockable room or office and carry some supplies with you. Do talk to your HR department and don't feel like you have to do it in the bathroom! Supplies might include:

- Handheld mirror to readjust yourself
- Small cooler with ice packs to store your milk
- Counter or shelf or table to put pump on
- Moist towel wipes to clean up
- Large tote bag or backpack to hold everything
- Curtains to put up if the room has windows for walls

When to pump depends on your supply and body. For me, I had to empty pretty regularly and found that this schedule worked:

- Nurse before leaving home: 8am
- Pump at work: 10am, 1pm, 4pm
- Nurse after getting back home: 6pm

PUMPING WHILE TRAVELING

Pumping while you're traveling away from home and your baby can be quite challenging even for the less modest, especially if you'll be spending long periods on the road or in the air. To smooth the way for yourself, do a little bit of research ahead of time:

- Read up on the latest airport security rules
  You will want your pump with you as a carry-on, so make sure you know what's allowed and not.
- Call and ask where you can pump
  The airport or conference center likely won't have a

designated place to do so discreetly, and some may point you toward public bathrooms. Make demands of conference organizers if you need to.

- Ask flight attendants about where to pump
  Likely, you'll end up staying in your seat or using a bathroom, but it's worth asking.
- Check if your hotel room comes with a fridge

And here are a few things to bring along:

- Extra pump batteries
  These are for when you don't have access to an outlet.
- Pump battery charger
- Usual pump and cleaning and storage supplies, plus a few extra
- Lots of water to drink on flights
- Antiseptic wipes
  For cleaning wherever you end up pumping.
- Insulated lunchbag/cooler
  For storing milk while you are away from a place with a fridge. Ice packs may not be allowed, so you can only store it for so long.
- Big poncho-like cover up
  In case you pump in a public or semi-public area, like an airport.

Chapter 13
Breast health issues

If you breastfeed or pump, health issues and pain are common but not ok. According to the survey, 9 out of 10 people who breastfeed run into one or more issues during the experience. It's tough!

Of those who have issues, the following chart shows how many people run into some of the more common problems. Some people may have more than one over the course of their whole breastfeeding experience.

Breast issue occurrence
FOR EVERY 10 WOMEN WHO PUMP OR BREASTFEED

engorgement	●	●	●	●	●	●	●	○	○	○
clogs	●	●	●	●	●	○	○	○	○	○
mastitis	●	●	●	○	○	○	○	○	○	○
thrush	●	●	○	○	○	○	○	○	○	○
baby tongue tie	●	○	○	○	○	○	○	○	○	○
low supply	●	●	○	○	○	○	○	○	○	○

Some other problems, like damaged nipples from barracuda babies and oversupply, are also not uncommon. Blebs and abscesses happen much less often, for about 1 in 100 new mamas who breastfeed or pump. Kellymom.com is a great resource for info on how to deal with these, though be aware that they're strong proponents of a certain type of parenting.

Make sure you are empty after each feeding or pumping once your body has settled into the groove. This is particularly important if you have oversupply or a baby that doesn't feed well, or are pumping exclusively. This will help prevent issues commonly related to poor drainage and dried milk in your ducts, like clogs, lumps, mastitis and, in some cases, abscesses (that was me, ouch). Below is a chart showing how common these types of problems are, according to the survey.

Breast issue co-occurrence related to poor drainage /oversupply
FOR EVERY 100 WOMEN WHO PUMP OR BREASTFEED

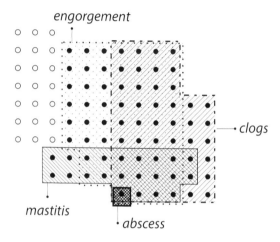

If you do have issues related to excess milk, learn how to manually express after each feeding. (Tip: it's easier to express into a large plastic container or bin and then pour the milk elsewhere, instead of trying to aim for a small bottle.) Break up any lumps or clogs right away. After the initial latching period, breastfeeding should NOT hurt, nor should anything you do to your breasts! Learn techniques from a lactation consultant, as you should never just squeeze at your breast, which can be painful and damaging.

Chapter 14
Weaning or reducing your milk output

If you need to stop for any reason, or if you were exclusively pumping and then switched to a breastfeeding baby that eats less, do it slowly! Do NOT go cold turkey (a breast surgeon unfamiliar with lactation actually gave me that exact instruction). Otherwise, you will get painful clogs, and lots of them.

A pump can be used to help you ease into the amount and frequency you want over time. For relief, some people swear by cold cabbage leaves or certain herbal teas, though that never worked for me. You can also ask your doctor for safe pain relief suggestions.

Chapter 15
Out and about

Get out and about! It's a great mood lifter and a good way to feel human and like your old self again.

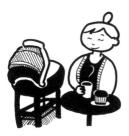

OUT WITH BABY

Small babies are incredibly portable, and they kind of lie there like a lump a lot of the time. Just pack up and head out. If you are nursing or if you have a bottle or two with you, you can spend quite a while outside. For formula drinkers, bring along pre-measured dry mix and a thermos bottle of warm water to make fresh milk on demand.

Here are a few suggestions that are mom- and baby-friendly:
- Mother-baby yoga or bootcamp (once you've healed enough to go)
- A walk down the street or to a park
- New mom groups
- Most restaurants
- Cafes where you can people-watch
- Sitting in a park with a magazine
- Vacation air travel
  You can do something fancy, like flying to Hawaii, or something heartwarming, like visiting beloved long-distance relatives. 1-3 months old is the easiest

time to travel with a child; it gets much more difficult between 4-16 months.

You'll want to look decent in public, but will still need to feed the baby if you're nursing. Bring along some washcloths or wipes to clean up if things get messy. Here are several outfit suggestions that minimize exposure, for those who are more modest, like me:

- T-shirt + nursing tank + cardigan on top
- Button-down + nursing tank on top
- Nursing cover + any nursing-friendly outfit that lets you access a boob

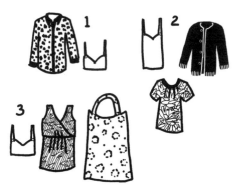

BABY-FREE

If you have someone who can watch the baby for an hour or two, you can also go out by yourself or with friends. Try things that you don't normally have a chance to do, that take time or solitude, like salons, bookstores, or shopping.

If you are breastfeeding, you will probably have about 2 hours free, depending on your supply. Nurse right before you head out the door to extend your time as long as possible. If your baby hasn't settled into a schedule yet, don't do anything that requires an appointment you may not be able to keep. You might leak during your excursion, so plan your outfit to ac-commodate that.

- Pick colors and patterns that obscure leaks.
  For example, choose black or busy dark prints over
  solid or pastel-colored clothing.
- Use disposable breast pads that stick on your bra.
  They are very thin and are amazing at preventing
  embarrassing wet spots! Washable ones made of
  organic natural materials totally did not do the job for
  me in public.

Chapter 16
The new normal

So what happens after things settle down with a newborn? Here are a few thoughts on what to expect.

FITTING IN YOUR OLD JEANS (OR NOT)

You might hear wildly different theories on how long it takes to get your old body back. Some claim it takes 9 months to make a baby, and another 9 months to get your body back. Or, breastfeeding proponents will tell you that you'll drop all that weight by nursing away the extra calories. Or, you might see celebrity magazines showing how actress X just dropped all her baby weight in 1 month.

Realistically, I think it just depends on genetics and your situation (and whether you have millions of dollars and a personal trainer in your home); the survey showed that individuals' experiences ranged across the board.

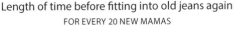

Length of time before fitting into old jeans again
FOR EVERY 20 NEW MAMAS

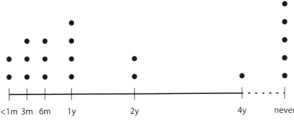

Some people's bodies snap right back, some change permanently (especially in the tummy and abdomen), and some discover their ribcage expanded temporarily. After giving birth, about 1 in 4 new moms find that their bodies changed permanently — they never fit into their old jeans again. And that's ok! Your body has done an amazingly difficult, life-changing thing, so be kind to yourself.

GOING BACK TO A WORKPLACE

If you're going back to work outside the home, it can be tough or liberating. How you feel about leaving the baby in someone else's care depends on your particular situation. (And also on all the crazy-making hormones running through your body.)

Just know that there's no winning with mommy guilt. Either you'll feel guilty for leaving the baby behind, or you'll feel guilty for not feeling guilty. You can ask your caretaker to send you pictures throughout the day, and that does help you stay connected. Going back to a workplace is a big change from being with your baby 'round the clock. You'll miss them for sure. But your brain gets really good at compartmentalizing, and it's very sweet to see your happy little baby again when you get home.

LIFE PARTNER RESPONSIBILITIES

You're both parents now, eek! You need to add childcare to your former shared household responsibilities.

Do make sure you both have the opportunity to have a break or some individual downtime during weekends. Here's a suggestion of how to split your tasks fairly, though it depends on your relationship and what you both prefer doing:

If one is at home, and partner is at a workplace.

The home person's entire day job is childcare. Do not expect any housework or dinner to get done because parenting young children is incredibly time consuming and hard to plan around.

Obviously, the workplace person's day job is at the workplace.

On "work days," housework and childcare need to be shared when both partners are at home. But given that the home person is spending a long day by themselves taking care of a baby, the workplace person should take over childcare in the mornings and evenings, while the home person makes meals and does dishes. During the weekends, you will both want a break from a long week of work, but share childcare and housework evenly.

If both partners work outside the home.
Split the childcare evenly between the two of you during at-home times. It's not fair to both your relationship and child if one person is providing all of the primary childcare and the other is out running store errands on weekends. During the week, try arranging your schedules so that one person goes to and leaves work early while the other goes and leaves late; this way, you minimize the cost of childcare and give the baby more bonding time with both of you.

• • • • •

Your schedule will change to accommodate your child's wake-up, hunger, and nap times. It helps to have other parent friends to hang out with; you may feel more at ease when there's a group understanding that you're all distracted, half-sane, and constantly being bossed around by baby needs. It can be challenging at first to make such a big change in your lifestyle, and while children grow and their needs change, you are now living your life with another human being as the priority. It will be challenging but fun. Once you get into a good groove, it's pretty amazing to watch your little baby grow and learn.

Chapter 17
After 6 weeks

Congratulations, you're a mom! You are amazing!

The first 6 weeks with a newborn are a crazy time in your life. All of the changes to your body and your life can be overwhelming. And, though it doesn't really ever end, it gets much better and much more sane. Hopefully, this book has prepared you for some of the bumps along the way. Like any other advice book, don't take anything you read here too seriously. Have faith in your own good sense.

Heal well, take good care of yourself, and enjoy your time with your cute new baby!

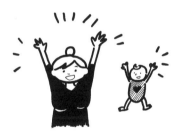

APPENDIX

Shopping list for you

None of these are must-haves. But many of them will make your life easier.

Post-birth healing
These are difficult to plan for, as you never know what may happen in the delivery room.
- Winged maxi pads of various strengths / a few adult diapers
- Donut pillow*
- Sitz bath*
- Ice packs / numbing spray / witch hazel pads
- Rinse bottle*
- Small pillow for incision*
- Stool softeners, check with doctor if breastfeeding
- Facial wipes

*Hospital may supply

Clothes
- High-waisted, comfy undies
- Whatever fits from 2nd and 3rd trimesters
- Yoga pants
- Bellyband

Feeding supplies
- Pillow
- Ergonomic chair with foot and armrests
- Small light-up analog clock
- Notepad and pen
- Entertainment viewable with one or no hands
  Ex: TV shows lined up on laptop, e-books, TV remote
- Many washcloths
- Dim lamp

Nursing clothes and supplies
- Nursing bras or camisoles
- Ribbed long tank tops
  Get ones that are super stretchy but fit to your body.
  Ex: Old Navy or Gap basics
- Zip-up sweatshirt with pockets but no hood
  Ex: fleece track jacket
- Reusable and washable fabric breast pads
- Disposable stick-on breast pads
- Loose button-up shirts that won't show wet spots easily
- Shirts and dresses made for nursing
- Nursing cover
- Nipple soothers and creams
  Ex: Motherlove, lanolin

Pumping supplies
- Pump
- The pump flange size that fits you
- Pump bottles
- Storage bags or containers for freezing
- Gallon zip-top bags or sterilizer bags
- Pumping bra
- For work: insulated lunch box, ice packs, containers

Food

- Hearty snacks
  Ex: string cheese, cookies, granola, trail mix, low-sodium jerky
- Water bottle that can be operated one-handed
- Emergency frozen meals
  Search the aisles for healthier options

Supplies for (avoiding) housecleaning

- Disposable dishware and silverware
- Paper towels and napkins
- Disposable surface wipes
  Ex: Clorox
- Disposable dusters and sweepers
  Ex: Swiffer

Things to prepare before birth

- Find delivery services you can use.
- Plan for helpers. If you have the budget, research and interview hired help.
- Make frozen meals – 2 to 4 weeks' worth of hot, nourishing food and soups
- If you normally wear contacts, make sure your glasses are an up-to-date prescription.
- Clean the pump and its accessories. Give it a trial run.
- Download books, movies, shows, and smartphone games. Resist the temptation to read /watch /play before the baby comes.
- Find a lactation consultant you like, if you plan on breastfeeding or pumping.

Household/caretaker help
- 0 – Friends and relatives stopping by to help (not visit)
- $ – Mother's helper
- $$ – Housekeeper
- $$$ – Post-partum doula
- $$$ – Part-time nanny
- $$$$ – Full-time nanny
- $$$$ – Full-time live-in nanny
- $$$$ – Night nanny

Customizable schedule

This is a way to help you get enough sleep and food by figuring out who does what. Don't actually try to put your newborn on a schedule; it's futile.

Useful average numbers for newborns:

- 10-12 feedings /day
- 20-40 minutes /feeding
- 10-12 diapers /day
- 11-18 hours total sleep /day
- 45-60 minutes /each time awake (includes feeding)

Things you can chart:
- Your sleep
- Your meals
- Your showers and bio breaks
- Feeding
- Diapering
- Holding the baby
- Cooking
- Chores and errands

	6am	7	8	9	10	11	Noon	1pm	2	3	4	5	6	7	8	9	10	11	Mid	1am	2	3	4	5
Baby																								
You																								

Additional survey-based charts and graphs

Delivery method for the first baby
(FOR EVERY 10 WOMEN)

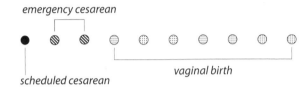

Help quality
How helpful were various forms of support?

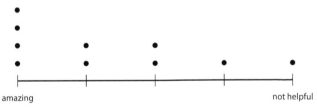

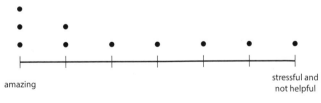

Mama mood in the first 6 weeks

Based on whether her situation is better than, worse than, or typical as compared to others' in the survey. It considers a combination of help, breastfeeding, birth issues, and sleep quality.

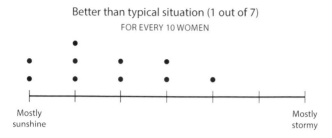

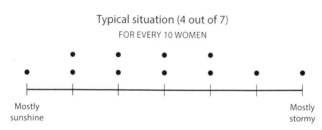

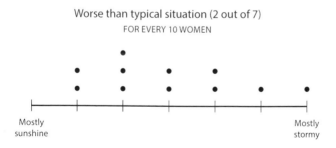

21013372R00047

Made in the USA
San Bernardino, CA
02 May 2015